SACRIFICE

SACRIFICE

Living life through Uranium, Coal, and School Buses
Loving life through My Son's Cerebral Palsy

WALTER WALDIE

XULON PRESS

Xulon Press
2301 Lucien Way #415
Maitland, FL 32751
407.339.4217
www.xulonpress.com

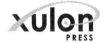

Paperback ISBN-13: 978-1-66287-682-0
Ebook ISBN-13: 978-1-66287-683-7

FOREWORD

I THINK I MET Rollie Waldie in 1967 or 1968, and as you'll read in this book, I was the Bobby Brittain who painted the trucks at Anderson Development. I didn't really get to know Rollie and his wonderful wife Judy until I became their pastor in 2003 at First Baptist Church of Thoreau, New Mexico. They used to invite my wife Judy and I, and some friends, for lunch on Sundays after church. That's where I got to know their son Lawrence, who has cerebral palsy. He loves to play football laying on the carpet, because he can't stand or sit by himself without help. But he loves to throw that soft football, and he loves the Dallas Cowboys.

As I read this book, I was reminded again of love in action. Rollie and Judy are two very talented people. I always knew (as their pastor and friend) that if we needed something, if something was broken or wouldn't work, they would help. Rollie could fix anything mechanical or build a new one that would work better. And Judy is a very bright lady with a willing and loving heart who can really cook. They are both exceptional people whose lives have been altered by Lawrence's disease. However, watching them love this young man is almost unbelievable. I'm convinced that it is Jesus Christ in them that gives them the power and strength to keep on, day after day, meeting the needs of a young man that would probably have died years ago without their loving care.

I enjoyed reading this book and learned many things that I hadn't known before about their story. I encourage anyone who knows Rollie and his family to read *Sacrifice*. First Corinthians 13:4-8 talks about what love really is. As you read this book, you'll see love (God's kind of love) lived through hard times and good times, as it challenges you to love like Jesus does.

Bobby J. Brittain, retired pastor and singer, still living in Grants, NM., who continues to fill in with sermon, support and song when needed.

INTRODUCTION

HELLO, MY NAME IS Rollie, and this is my life story. While growing up in Silver City, New Mexico, I started having lots of exciting experiences biking, hunting, swimming, and riding horses. I was fortunate to go with my dad, Red Waldie, occasionally on short trips hauling cattle, running heavy equipment, gravel for roads and watch him operate the truck, loader and dozer. I was in my pre-teens when I started learning how to drive big trucks and heavy equipment.

After moving to Grants, New Mexico, the uranium capital of the world, dad became the supervisor of Anderson Development Corporation. This trucking company hauled uranium ore for Kerr-McGee Mill in Ambrosia Lake, where I lived with my parents, attended elementary school, and would later earn my first paycheck. The Ambrosia Lake land that dad leased was his chance to start a 250-acre alfalfa farm and live out his dream of raising cattle and horses.

I was in my twenties when Maxie Anderson took over as the owner of the trucking company, after his dad Carl Anderson retired. Maxie asked me if I would supervise a job in Waco, Texas. The job involved hiring a crew to remove the copper and water valves from the steam-powered generation station that provided electricity for Waco and the surrounding communities.

After returning to New Mexico from the job in Waco, I worked through the winter in Ambrosia Lake at the trucking company; and again,

Maxie asked me to supervise a job, this time in Natchez, Mississippi. The Mississippi River ran beside the land and was separated by a tall levy. I would plant the old farm and fence it into many pastures so yearling calves could graze.

The next job I had was supervising Red Rock Transportation Company, a school bus operation that Maxie Anderson, my dad, and Carl Lytle, a friend that lived in Ambrosia Lake had purchased. The one hundred bus routes were in McKinley County and San Juan County, New Mexico, and this job would keep me busy for the next six years.

After the school bus business was sold, I purchased a truck and trailer and started hauling uranium ore. While I was an owner operator, Judy Barton, with her son Jeremy, and I were married and started our lives living in Thoreau New Mexico. While living and working in this little town, a special child came into our lives.

After working for Kerr-McGee until their final days of operation, Santa Fe Coal Company hired me. I worked for them in maintenance and had some tough interactions with one of the bosses from my first day. I would be challenged on every move I made, but I eventually lived through the pressure and became a maintenance foreman. A few years later, I became the heavy equipment coordinator.

As I grew older, another quiet danger was slowly starting to emerge in my life. Diabetes tried to take me down. My A1C had climbed to double digits, but I refused the new suggested meds and declared war on diabetes that day. After three months had passed, my doctor entered the exam room with a smile and handed me the test results that showed I was no longer diabetic, but that test result did not mean the hard work was over. After seventy years of bad eating habits, I had to replace everything. Food that was low in carbs, no more cereal and sweets, I had to develop my own new diet.

TABLE OF CONTENTS

WHERE IT ALL STARTED

I GREW UP IN Silver City, New Mexico, where my dad, Red Waldie, who owned his truck and trailers and hauled everything he could to provide for his family. Sometimes when dad let me ride with him and we would not be back until after lunch, mom would make me a lunch, too. I was not a teenager yet when I began learning to work and have responsibilities. Dad let me operate my Uncle Dave's D-6 dozer at the ranch, while he was cleaning out an old dirt dam to catch water. He would let me move his truck around the backyard when he was doing maintenance, fixing flat tires, and greasing the truck.

Out at the ranch where my mom grew up, there was a big, thirty-foot-wide by fifty-foot-long and twelve-foot-deep irrigation pool that held enough water to irrigate all the fields in the little valley below. The windmill on top of the ridge pumped the water that filled the pool, and the pool had some goldfish that lived in it for years. They were about eight inches long and swam around slowly, teasing us as we tried to catch them by hand. My cousin Rich and I would go swimming every chance we could in that pool.

I was always in the middle of everything while growing up, trying to help. There at the ranch, I first learned how to feed and milk the Guernsey milk cow, which would become one of my chores later in my life. I helped gather and corral the cattle with my dad and Uncle Dave, so the calves could be branded, get their ear tags, and get vaccinated. The bigger calves would be weaned off from their mothers and kept separated in another pasture. I also learned where our meat came from when my dad and uncle butchered the ranch's steer, which was what had to be done if you were to survive on a ranch. I was fortunate that mom and dad allowed me to see and learn how to do these things in my childhood.

While I was growing up, mom decided she wanted to paint the inside of the house and asked dad to take her to the hardware store to pick out the paint color. While they were there, the owner of the store, who was a friend of dad's, persuaded my dad to try out his new spray gun. He told him it would cut the time in half for painting; well, that was music to dad's ears. Mom and dad came home with the paint gun, the paint, and very little knowledge about using a paint gun. Dad did not have a regulator to control the air pressure but connected the paint gun to his compressor without one and began painting.

When he finally finished painting the inside of the house, over-spraying everything, mom told dad to get rid of the paint sprayer. Dad was just trying to get done so he could get back to his other jobs, not knowing the paint gun would cost him a lot more time cleaning everything that should not have been painted than saving him time. Painting was never dad's favorite thing to do after that.

When I was older, and we were living in Milan, New Mexico, mom and dad would take me to Silver City in the summer to visit with my aunt Helen, who I called Ammie, and my cousin Rich. Ammie took me under her wing and made sure I always had things to do and did not get sick. If any of us felt bad or had a runny nose, she would give us all a penicillin shot. One time, she quietly prepared the first shot for Rich, who was horrified by needles. He ran into the master bedroom and dove under the bed, grabbing hold of the far corner bed leg and not letting go. After seeing my cousin finally get his shot, I was sure I did not want one, but Ammie knew if I caused a problem, I would have a bigger problem from my parents when I got home. Well, it was my turn, so I surrendered and got my shot. I remember saying to myself how glad I am that mom doesn't do this at home.

During those summers, Rich and I would ride bicycles from Ammie's house in Silver City to the ranch. There was never any problems or dangers back then, and everyone driving on the roads waved to each other when they met. Riding the eight miles out to the ranch on bikes was a challenge, going up and down hills on the highway until we reached the turn-off from the highway, and then riding three miles on the rutted dirt road. It would be another year until Rich and his sister Barbara got Honda trail bikes, which changed everything. The next year, we were gas-powered and could ride through town and up the hills to the ranch in no time.

OUR FIRST MOVE TO SOCORRO, NEW MEXICO

DAD, WHO ALREADY OWNED a truck, got a job hauling copper from a small mine in Socorro, New Mexico. Once he got his living arrangements set up at the mine site, he brought us there to stay for a week. We were miles out of town in the worst heat we ever had in New Mexico. I went exploring and was shocked by the extreme surroundings around the mine. On all the hills and in the ditches around the mine, everything was covered with round rocks, cactus, and rattlesnakes. With all the snakes everywhere, I was not wandering off far. So, I spent my time around the mine site, helping anybody that would let me.

Every day, the equipment had to be greased and checked for oil and coolant levels. Everything was fueled up, checked for flat tires, and inspected for snakes that crawled everywhere after dark. They were in the wheel wells and against the shaded side of the tires. You quickly learned to check where you put your hands. The doors were kept shut on all the equipment at night. Dad said while he was driving, if he started thinking about snakes, he would have to pull over and stop the truck to check out the cab. Every day, dad would see a rattlesnake around the ore pile while he was loading the truck or see one in the truck's mirrors, hanging over the side of the dump trailer as he was headed to the stockpile. There had to be a rattlesnake den there somewhere in the mine.

A friend at the mine told dad he had stocked a dirt pond with fish on his ranch, and we could go fishing there sometime. Dad had never taken us fishing before, so this would be our first time. I had visions of catching lots of fish. He bought us fishing poles, worms, and salmon eggs, and away we went. It took us a while to find the pond, but as soon as we did, we started setting up our poles. I was not as brave as I thought when I had to touch that worm and put it on my hook, but I finally manned up and started fishing.

I could tell that dad had little patience for fishing, but he sat there under a tree, trying to catch a fish like the rest of us. Even though dad never mentioned it, we knew that he would be working into the night once our fishing trip was over to get things ready for work in the morning. We all sat fishing patiently for a couple of hours, waiting for a fish to bite. Dad kept getting more impatient until finally he just could not sit any longer. He told us that he did not think the fish were going to start biting until the sun went down and it cooled off. We all decided, for dad's sake, to go home and come back another day when it was cooler; that was the last time I ever went fishing with my dad. After a few months, the little mine shut down, which would put dad out of work. But this time, uranium had been discovered north of Grants, New Mexico, so there were possible opportunities for his trucking business.

Chapter 3

GRANTS, NEW MEXICO: THE URANIUM CAPITAL OF THE WORLD

AMBROSIA LAKE WAS A flat valley that used to have a shallow, natural lake where an old stagecoach stop was built. The lake had been dried up for sixty years, and many tourists are still driving there in search of a fishing paradise because the signs on old Route 66 still point north to Ambrosia Lake. The discovery of uranium in Ambrosia Lake started a huge boom in the region. In 1962 Kermac Nuclear Fuels would merge into Kerr-McGee Corp and build the uranium mill in Ambrosia Lake. It would be years before the mines were all built and the thousands of workers that came looking for an opportunity would be employed. Grants and the surrounding towns were called the "Uranium Capital of the World." It was a busy time, with houses, motels and restaurants being built in Grants and Gallup. Uranium claims were being staked in and around Ambrosia Lake, as people were trying to get land that was worth mining. Miners and workers were coming for work and finding places to live from all around the country. They settled in Grants, Gallup, and the surrounding towns; some of them bought trailer houses and moved into a trailer park in Ambrosia Lake. There was even an elementary school and a cafe built in Ambrosia Lake.

The government was buying all the enriched uranium that was produced to make nuclear weapons to be used as America's deterrent against the aggression of the Soviet Union. America was finding itself in a dangerous cold war.

Dad got his next trucking job hauling uranium ore for Calumet and Hecla's incline mine north of Grants toward San Mateo. He had to purchase another truck and a new caterpillar side dump loader to load them, and the ore was hauled to Homestake Mill. There were now three uranium mills in the area: Kerr-McGee in Ambrosia Lake; Homestake, three miles north of Milan; and Anaconda, east of Bluewater Village and west of Grants. Homestake Mill started milling ore from small independent mines until their mines started producing.

Kerr-McGee and Homestake were continuing their exploration work in search of new ore bodies, where new mine shafts would later be established. Anaconda's ore was delivered by train from the Jack Pile mine in Paguate, New Mexico, which was the world's largest open-pit uranium mine at that time. When Calumet and Hecla mine shut down, however, dad would be out of work again.

As Homestake's mines started stockpiling their ore, the mill was looking for a contractor to haul the ore for them. They gave dad the contract to haul their ore until they purchased their own fleet of trucks. Dad had to buy some more trucks to haul the amount of ore the three mines were producing.

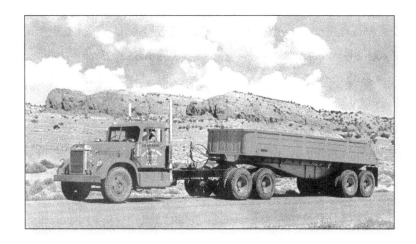

Hauling uranium ore to Homestake Mill

About eighteen months after dad started hauling Homestake's ore, they started buying their own fleet of trucks. Homestake was still mining and milling uranium ore when the downfall of the uranium industry happened on July 16, 1979. Ironically, dad was the first trucking company to haul Homestake's uranium ore, and, in the end, I scraped the ore pads and hauled the last of their ore when the miners removed the stopes. (Stopes are big sections of the ore body that are left untouched to support and keep the mined-out, unsupported areas around them from caving in.)

Dad was aware that this layoff was going to happen, and he had already been asked to supervise Anderson Development Corporation, who hauled the ore for Kerr-McGee Corporation. He supervised the company trucks, while using his trucks to keep up with the hungry mill until more company trucks were purchased. Our family moved to Ambrosia Lake in 1958 and into a trailer house in the trucking company's yard, where we would live for the next eighteen years.

Now that my family was living a normal life again, I rode a school bus for the first time to the elementary school a mile away. This was the time in America when we were learning what to do if a nuclear bomb detonated, and we were exposed to nuclear fallout. We practiced drills at school, like getting under our desks and bowing our heads down, as well as being given handouts to take home and read with our parents about the importance of building a fallout shelter and storing survival supplies. We built a corral and barn, planting ten acres around them. We grew a garden and grazed dad's horses and milk cow on the pasture.

My desire to learn how to operate the heavy equipment came from being around my dad and the workers, hearing the stories they told about their experiences. I was fifteen years old when I operated a D-8 dozer that stacked the ore on the ore pads for the loaders as they loaded the trucks. I also operated the road grader to repair the gravel haul roads. After I turned seventeen, I was finally earning a paycheck, working for $1.55 an hour. I was getting very wealthy at this rate because I was living with my parents and working evenings after school and on most weekends. I remember driving with my best friend Johnny Bell when he opened the glovebox on my 1967 Ford Mustang and counted six uncashed paychecks in it.

During this time in America, the Cold War was raging. Our government was desperate for the uranium mills to enrich the uranium ore into yellow cake, which they were buying to build the nuclear arsenal that would counter the aggressive actions of the USSR. Because of the importance of mining the uranium, for the security of our country, the name "Cold War Patriots" was given to all the uranium miners, mill workers, and truck drivers that worked in this dangerous environment for years.

We lived in Ambrosia Lake on section 30 in the trucking yard, across the highway from section 30 west mine site. The truck yard was a half mile north of the Kerr-McGee Uranium Mill. Our drinking water well was in the middle of the uranium ore deposit, and the radioactive mine water, discharged from section 30 west mine, ran under the road to our corrals and

9

vegetable garden and irrigated our pasture, where our chickens, milk cow and calf, and horses would graze. No one knew about the damage to your health this was causing.

The trucking company did all the work for the mill, including building the drill sites and roads for the exploration drill rigs, building all the new haul roads to the new mine sites, and leveling and compacting all the truck loads of waste to make the ore pads. As the uranium ore was hoisted from the mine, the ore was dumped on the pads, pushed up in piles, and loaded and hauled to the mill. Sometimes the mill's loaders would be out of service, so I would take one of our loaders and feed the ore into the grizzly that fed the plant. I was lucky in my life to get to operate all the equipment that the company owned, and I would keep using this experience the rest of my life. I was doing all the specialty jobs that were needed. When a situation came up where a dozer was needed somewhere to help fix or build something, I would load a dozer on the lowboy (a heavy built flat trailer with 3 tandem axles hooked to a big diesel truck), and I would haul it where it was needed to do the job, I would do the job myself and then take everything back home.

The company purchased a link-belt track machine with a cable-controlled backhoe, mounted where the boom was on the 30-ton link belt crane. It was acquired to clean out the drilling mud ponds, where the two modified oil field drill rigs were drilling the section 19 mine shaft. These two coupled drill rigs used a very big drill bit to make a ten-foot diameter hole and lower the prefabbed shaft sections, making it the first mine shaft sunk in New Mexico by drilling. I maintained and operated the backhoe for a few months before an operator was hired to take my place.

On my normal workday, my job was loading the uranium ore onto the trucks or pushing up big piles with the dozer, making more room on the ore pads or driving a haul truck. I also spent time helping mechanics repair the trucks, loaders, and dozers. I was fortunate to learn from different mechanics while they made the major repairs, which was another opportunity for me to learn about the importance of maintenance in keeping everything running.

However, the government at that time was not very forthright about the dangers everyone was exposed to with the radiation. Many miners, truck drivers, and mill workers had died from radiation exposure over the years, and there are still a lot of us that are fighting the effects of it today. The Department of Labor finally started compensating people that could prove they were exposed and worked in the mills or mines or hauled the uranium during the time the government was buying the yellow cake. This exposure would eventually be the source of my dad's lung problems and my lung damage as well. Because of the normally hot weather in New Mexico and air conditioners not being around yet, the truck drivers and equipment operators kept their windows open, which allowed the radioactive dust to blow in their faces and be breathed in. Inhaling the dried dust particles and drinking the water were major reasons for the workers' exposure.

Years after retirement from the mills, mines, and trucking jobs, when the workers were dealing with many respiratory problems, there was little to no information about compensating them. The only way of learning about the program was from having a chance encounter with an old mining friend, who was also suffering from the radiation effects but was being compensated and told people about it. Our government, which was so desperate to buy all the yellow cake being produced, regardless of the dangers at that time, did not advertise the way they should have to find and help the radiation-exposed workers that were responsible for producing the yellow cake in the first place.

During this time, when health problems were being contributed to uranium exposure, many people were overlooked, like my mom. She lived and worked in the truckyard, drank the same water, and breathed the same air at the trucking company for eighteen years. She worked every day for free for dad's sake, doing all the secretary work, payroll, billing, and purchasing for the trucking company. Since she was never on the payroll, she was not eligible for the compensation given to the paid workers for the radiation exposure. Sometimes the good people that are trying to help do not matter to others.

One day, our boss, Carl Anderson, came out to visit and look things over. When he saw the D-8 dozers working in the winter without any cabs, he called them "prairie schooners" and they were very embarrassing to him. What a great observation, as we had been trying to get him to buy the cabs for years. We installed two, big two-inch diameter cables that were bent to make arches on each side of the dozers; then a tarp was tied to the cables, protecting the operator from rain and snow. Carl got so wound up about it that he told dad to order the cabs for the dozers and get all the old trucks painted. The cabs got ordered, but the mechanic that could paint the trucks was in the hospital, so it was going to take some time to get that done.

After a week went by, one of the truck drivers named Bob Brittain asked my dad if he was not needed to haul ore for a few days, could he paint his truck. Dad was excited about someone wanting to paint their truck that he agreed to schedule the paint job. Bob could take his time and not be in a hurry. When he finished cleaning, sanding, and painting, he removed the masking paper and had dad come and inspect the job. Dad was so impressed with the paint job that he asked Bob to paint the rest of the trucks. No one knew at that time that the radiation danger in the dust particles were in all the office and maintenance jobs, cleaning and sanding the old trucks that had years of uranium dust in the frames and inside the cabs and engine compartments, which fell to the shop floor, only to be swept up, breathed in and dumped outside. Unaware workers, mechanics, painters, office workers, and visitors that would come onto the truck yards, mines, and mill sites were breathing the dust in while they were doing their jobs, not knowing the damage it was doing.

In 1983 Kerr-McGee would become Quivera Mining Corporation and would continue the leaching and reclamation work in Ambrosia Lake.

Chapter 4

THE URANIUM CAPITAL BI-COUNTY FAIR

WHEN I REACHED MY junior high school years, I became friends with all the kids that came with their parents to the square dances. Ted Garroute, a good friend, would come and call or sing out the dance movements to the music, and everyone would grab a partner and join in the dances. These square dances were being held all over the state and once a year, there was a big gathering for square dancing in Albuquerque.

A lot of the adults that were square dancing became the founding members of the Uranium Capital Bi-County Fair Association. Their goal was to buy some land and build a fairground where all the kids in Cibola and McKinley Counties could compete locally, instead of having to drive eighty miles to the Valencia County Fair in Belen, New Mexico. Everyone knew we needed a local fair, but now it needed to be built.

A good friend of dad's donated the land in Prewitt, New Mexico, and I hauled a D8 caterpillar dozer, with a carry-all scraper coupled to it, to the new property and leveled the land. The fair board members decided on the layout, and people came to help; some only brought a hammer or pliers, but they showed up and volunteered. I hauled the buildings from Ambrosia Lake that were donated to the fairgrounds by Kerr-McGee. These buildings had to have offices and display booths built inside them, as well as plumbing for the water and sewer systems. I remember all the many smashed and cut fingers from all the boys and girls that were helping nail the tin over the stalls as the fairgrounds were being built.

The Prewitt Rodeo Club started building the new rodeo grounds with big bleachers, for the fair. The Rodeo Club members and the community came together to support the fair with their purchases of the animals that made it to the sale.

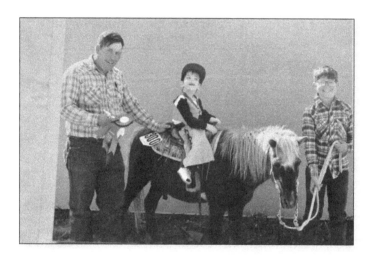

Lawrence winning lead line event at Uranium Capital Bi-County Fair

The bleachers were donated from the Gallup Indian Ceremonials and many welders with their welding rigs donated their time to cut apart the bleachers into sections. These pieces of bleachers were hauled from Gallup to Prewitt by local truckers who donated their trucks, fuel, and time to help. It took us two months to set all the pillars in place and pour the cement floor, and then start assembling the bleachers.

I can remember when the rough stock pins for the rodeo grounds were built. Welding trucks were scattered around the arena, with their welders running, cutting, and welding pipe for days. My dad and Lawrence Elkins had just finished the pin they were working on and were ready to drive out when they realized they had welded themselves in. After all the laughs and jokes from everybody there, they had to cut out the panel they had just finished to free their truck. All the work done on the fair and rodeo grounds was accomplished by a great bunch of friends that enjoyed working together until the project was finished.

It was under these bleachers where kids from all around the two counties would come to dance to the western music and enjoy life.

Chapter 5

RANCHING AND FARMING

AFTER WE MOVED TO Ambrosia Lake, dad's dream of ranching and farming came true. He leased many sections of land over the years and grew a nice herd of cattle and some good horses. We spent many weekends building corrals, fences, and dirt tanks. We prepared a half-section of farmland and planted alfalfa. These two life dreams of dad's were finally coming true.

We bought seven quarter mile long side roll irrigation systems and two miles of twelve-inch mainline pipe to transport the water. We used an old 1965 B model Mack truck with a 5 and 4 transmission and installed a 1200-gal per minute pump in the frame to provide the side roll systems with enough pressured water to irrigate everything. The old truck would idle as it pumped the water, and when we had to shut down some of the side rolls for cutting or bailing, we just shifted the transmission in the old Mack to a lower gear and kept on irrigating. We bought all the equipment needed to grow and sell the hay also. We bought a Heston two wire baler, a Heston 420 riding swather to cut the hay, a rake to dry the hay, a 7520 John Deere tractor with a 25' wide folding disk, a 3020 John Deere tractor for planting cutting and bailing, a twelve foot wide Brillion planter and a New Holland 160 bale stacker wagon to pick up deliver and stack the hay.

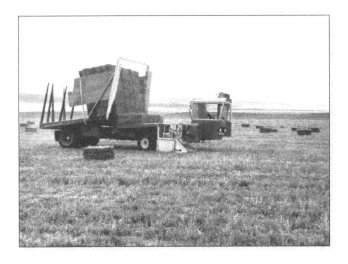

Loading bales of hay in alfalfa field

The ranches that got the hay delivered by the stacker wagon loved it, because it made their stack for them. The cement pad I stacked the hay on was once the floor of a big shop. I dug a fifteen-foot-deep and one-hundred-foot-long trench beside the concrete pad with our loader. I backed my truck and flatbed trailer into it and loaded the hay on the trailer, I dropped the bales from the stacks on the concrete pad down on the trailer and as close to where they should be so the two helpers could move them to their spot. The usual way to load hay on a forty-foot float took several men to buck the bales up five feet from the field and onto the trailer, then a few more men to lift them from the trailer as the stack grew higher and the truck and trailer had to keep driving up the row of bales in the field. Our design was less physically demanding, where my two workers and I could load 450 bales in an hour and thirty minutes. Dad was still living out his life dreams working cattle and growing alfalfa when he died. My dad also had damaged lungs from all the radiation exposure. He never knew about the government program to help the miners before he died in his sleep in 1993.

Chapter 6

MOTHER'S POEMS

MY MOTHER HAD ALWAYS been the backbone of our family, constantly adjusting her day to the changing events that happened on a ranch but always there with a hot meal when we gathered cattle. One time, when we were branding calves, she brought a pressure cooker full of pinto beans and cornbread. She told dad the beans needed to be warmed up, to which dad said he could do that. He took her pressure cooker with the top off, so the beans could be stirred, and balanced the pot of beans on the round top of the branding pig. The handle of the pot was resting on a small piece of wood that he stood up against the side of the branding pig. We were licking our chops and watching the pot when suddenly the plastic handle melted and the pot of beans fell, spilling half of them onto the ground.

There we were, with no heavy gloves to grab the hot pot that now had no handle. Dad stuck a branding iron inside the pot, leveling it, and, with the other branding iron, drug the pot away from the pig, saving half the beans. Well, those beans sure tasted good, even with knowing what the branding iron was just used for.

While mom waited for us to finish irrigating the alfalfa, herding cattle, branding calves, or building fence, she would use the time to write her poems. Mom had stacks of notebooks filled with her poems. She would write poems about how God's Word would always make her see things that really mattered in life. Mom also wrote poems about everyone in the family (even the horses and dogs), the weather with the rain and the snow, and all the exciting events that had happened in her lifetime. She would always present her new grandchildren with a special poem, written for each one.

Mom finally got to attend a big poetry convention in Denver, where all the famous authors she had heard about were reciting their poems for people. Mom continued writing poetry and attending church with Judy, Lawrence, and I until she passed away on December 4th, 2014.

I GOT TO SEE GOD'S FIRST MIRACLE IN MY LIFE

DURING MY TIME WORKING at the trucking company, I found myself involved in a terrible accident and quickly learned what miracles Jesus can perform. I started the day driving a Peterbilt truck with a three-axle trailer, hauling a piece of ten-foot-diameter by thirty-foot-long pipe to Church Rock mine, where it was used as a culvert in a big ditch. After unloading the pipe at the mine, I started back home and was halfway back when tragedy happened.

I was driving past Prewitt, New Mexico, on the interstate, and it began raining as a passenger bus loaded with people started passing me. The bus and I made our way on the wet road going downhill and were making a right turn. The passenger bus was about two-thirds of the way past me at this point. In this part of the interstate, the highway department had left the median undeveloped, with the high bench of lava rock still untouched for a mile. As the big lava median started tapering down, we could see cars stopped on the opposite side of the interstate. The truck and bus brakes were applied at the same time and as we came out of the right turn, we saw our side of the interstate with cars stopped on the right shoulder, all because of an earlier accident down in the median.

We were both sliding at the same speed when we both saw a car stopped in the passing lane looking down into the median at the original accident. This driver was completely unaware of the dangerous situation she had caused. As the passenger bus with its brakes locked was about to hit the car, the driver in the car took notice, turned right, and drove broadside in front of me. I had no place to go, with cars parked on the right side shoulder beside me and the bus still sliding on my left side. The truck hit the car and climbed over it, and the car was sliding under the truck in front of my right-side tractor tires.

The car was being torn apart from the friction of the highway; the woman and the small boy were sitting on the driver's seat, sliding along in front of the truck tires. The truck started turning toward the line of cars on the right side of the road. I was headed toward an open spot where a car had left the scene. The next car past the open spot was hit on the trunk by the truck's left front steering tire, and then the truck hit the curb and went down the embankment, off the road. The turn the truck made after hitting the parked car caused the trailer to slide, pulling the truck away from the driver's seat that the woman and the boy were on, leaving them on the seat in the road as the trailer followed the truck through the right-away fence. Somehow, the woman and boy were both alive.

After the truck's left front tire hit the back of the parked car, the back glass broke, and a piece of glass cut the baby's leg that was sleeping in the back seat. The passenger bus that was still sliding beside me during the wreck stopped and was able to unload its passengers. The bus driver and the stunned passengers walked out to where the truck stopped and told me they witnessed the entire accident. When the wrecker arrived at the scene, there was nothing left for it to haul. He had to get a small flatbed trailer to load all the pieces of the first car. Somebody should have gone back to slow the traffic down and prevent this accident from happening.

The next day, I returned to the wreck site and repaired the bent tie rod, replaced the cross-over fuel line, and helped fix the broken right-away fence before driving the truck back home. If I had refused to deal with what happened, I might have quit driving trucks forever. It is just natural for people that have been involved in tragic events in their lives to never want to repeat them. To this day, I am extra careful of the dangers that we face on the roads.

It is only because of Jesus that no one was killed.

Chapter 8

JO-JO THE SPIDER MONKEY

A FUNNY STORY TO share while living at Anderson Development Corporation. Carl Anderson's secretary, in Albuquerque, called dad and asked if she could give him her spider monkey Jo-Jo. Dad could not tell her no, so she loaded up Jo-Jo and brought him out to Ambrosia Lake. After a while of trying to live with Jo-Jo, we eventually found out why she had to get rid of him. He stayed in our trailer house in an empty bedroom, with his ten-foot-long chain hooked on the doorknob. He was ornery and did not have a good relationship with anybody. Sometimes he was let outside, with his chain still on.

Our first bad day with Jo-Jo started when mom came into the living room where Jo-Jo was hanging out on the back of a chair. He jumped across the room onto mom's arm, biting deeply into her hand. He would not let go and was swinging from her hand with his sharp teeth dug in. Mom's hand was bleeding badly, and she screamed but could not free her hand from Jo-Jo. I ran into the room and saw him hanging from her hand, as she stood, frozen in shock, in the middle of the living room. I kicked Jo-Jo like a football off my mom. He slammed against the ceiling, and his lifeless body fell to the floor. I unhooked his chain from the doorknob and carried him outside, tied his chain to the yard fence, and laid him on the lawn.

Everybody in the truck yard heard the screams in our home, and dad came running from the shop, saw what had happened, and hurried mom to the doctor in Grants for a tetanus shot, some pain pills, and a big bandage on her hand. Jo-Jo was now an outside spider monkey.

My cousins Jenny and Susie came up from Silver City to visit us. Well, you guessed it, we forgot to get Jo-Jo's permission. Jo-Jo did not like to be around people and, even worse, a bunch of people. This was one of Jo-Jo's bad days, and he was really upset at the dogs that were laying in the grass a little too close to his area. He thought all the yard was his, so he was mad. The noise from the dogs barking and Jo-Jo screaming drew all of us kids into the yard. Jo-Jo had managed to unlatch his chain and was still holding it in his hand, as if it were hooked. He was planning to get some revenge on the dogs, but when Susie and Jenny ran into the yard to see what all the commotion was, Jo-Jo found new victims. He threw the chain down and jumped on Susie, wrapping his arms around her waist and began biting her on her belly. Screams and shouts were heard all around the place. Mechanics and office workers came running to see what was happening. Jo-Jo was screaming also, with his mouth open and snapping his sharp teeth. He jumped down on the grass and began chasing everybody. Finally, with gloves on, we caught the monkey and the chaos ended, though Susie still thinks she could hear me laughing at her. Well, I hope I wasn't laughing but there was sure some quick scrambling to get behind somebody to hide from that monkey. Now Jo-Jo had lost all privileges and was being sent to prison in the truck shop.

Dad decided that we could not continue fighting Jo-Jo, so he put the monkey upstairs in the shop and told everyone to leave him alone; and if you needed something from the storage room, make sure he was chained up. Now he was alone in the storage room, where he still messed with anyone that came in. The only safe way to go up there was wearing welding gloves and to never tease him or turn your back on him.

One time, a mechanic went upstairs to get a bundle of shop rags and forgot to shut the door. Later in the day, there was a loud bang in the shop. Jo-Jo had dragged a big light bulb out of the door and was waiting to drop it on someone. The same mechanic that left the door open was standing under the stairs, shouting at the monkey. When we all got there, we saw the light bulb broken on the floor, and Jo-Jo was looking down screaming at us. Jo-Jo did not realize it then, but he was going to have much better days ahead of him.

Kerr-McGee hired a security guard named Gus Raney. Gus was a tough, old man that grew up in the twenties in the Silver City and Cliff areas in southwest New Mexico. Back in those days, disagreements were often settled with guns. Gus had become a deputy marshal in his younger days and had helped catch some bad guys. He was cautious of everyone, and he and his wife carried handguns wherever they were. They also had several mean guard dogs that would bite you, so you did not visit them unless they knew you were coming.

Kerr-McGee, with Dad's help, hired Gus to protect all their mining claims. The uranium company had hundreds of claims spread for miles around the county. Gus was given a four-wheel drive Bronco to drive around and check the claims. Gus kept all his supplies, food, water, clothing, tent, and his dogs inside the Bronco. He came to the truck yard to gas up and leave his weekly report on the claims; this was his only opportunity to visit with people. He always brought drawings he made of strange things, like Bigfoot and the very strange spaceships of varying shapes and sizes, that were flying around the top of Mount Taylor. He explained what each spaceship was doing and where they landed. Gus had quite an imagination, but we never discovered if anything was true. We did not have a scanner to copy the hand drawn pictures and Gus would not let us keep them. We all were really impressed with his stories.

Gus called dad one afternoon and told him the Bronco would not start. It had been raining, and the roads were a muddy mess. Dad told me to get the utility truck checked out and take Harold Platero, a friend and loader operator, with me to go rescue Gus. We both had worked all day but were up to the challenge. With the directions Gus had given us, we set off.

First, we drove to the grocery store in Milan and bought food supplies before heading out. The utility truck was the roughest riding truck on the old dirt roads that we ever rode in. It took us a while to find Gus, who was several miles east of Mount Taylor; it was midnight when we finally got there.

We hooked the Bronco up to our utility truck with a tow beam and started back home. The utility truck had a single seat cab, and it was crowded.

We drove quietly for a while when a jackrabbit ran in front of us. Gus said, "Stop, I need that rabbit for my dogs." I stopped, and Gus got out and shot the rabbit. He walked over, picked it up, and threw it inside the Bronco with his dogs. We drove a while longer and stopped to fix a sandwich. Harold reached down on the floorboard to get our box with the food. When he reached inside the box, he discovered that Gus had been spitting his tobacco in the box. The tobacco spit had covered everything inside; well, that instantly stopped our hunger pains.

We made it back to the truck yard at daybreak, and the day shift workers came outside to see what was happening. I parked the truck, and the men began looking everything over. They saw the mess the dogs had made with their supper and started teasing the mechanics that would be repairing it. After Gus removed his things and the dogs from the Bronco, the mechanics had to steam clean inside and outside before they would start the repairs to the truck.

After this adventure, mom and dad came up with an idea to get rid of Jo-Jo. They asked Gus if he would like to have Jo-Jo. Gus said he would enjoy the monkey's company while he was out alone for weeks at a time. That new partnership was appreciated by both, as they became fast friends, and Jo-Jo would ride in Gus's lap as he drove down the road and pick through Gus's beard.

The last time we heard about Gus and Jo-Jo, they were stopped at a gas station in Grants fueling up. Gus was inside talking with the owner while the attendant was fueling up the Bronco. The young boy suddenly noticed something moving through the side glass. Jo-Jo had pulled Gus's revolver from its holster on the steering wheel and onto the seat and was trying to pick it up. The young attendant stopped what he was doing and ran into the store to tell his boss, but Gus told the boy it was alright because there was no bullet in the barrel. Jo-Jo and Gus were together for years.

THAT POWER POLE

THE TRUCKING COMPANY PURCHASED an old cable-controlled carry-all that was pulled with a D8 cable dozer. This machine was used to move a lot of dirt when building new haul roads. It was my job to get the carry-all set up.

I connected the dozer's cables to the carry-all and started adjusting the brakes, which would hold the heavy load up while the carry-all transported the material. When the load was ready to dump, another control arm was pulled, raising up the front gate and pulling the end gate forward dumping all the material. I was going up and down the fence line on the outside of the truck yard, loading, dumping, and adjusting again for a couple of hours. I was leaning over the back of the dozer, watching the brakes, when I heard this crunching noise. I turned around and saw the dozer blade had hit the power pole three feet above the ground right in the middle of the dozer blade, I heard arching from above as I stopped the dozer. The pole was broken and was swinging from the wires, finally swinging out a few feet from its broken base. The sudden movement of the pole had caused the wires to touch, tripping the fuses on the power line.

The electricians from the mill ran down and drilled a hole beside the broken stub and installed a fifteen-foot pole beside it, tying the swinging pole to it with many straps. The power line was energized in a couple of hours, and the broken pole was replaced with a new one the following weekend. I continued fine-tuning the brakes and had them ready to work by the end of shift.

It was about this time that Carl Anderson retired, and his son Maxie took over ownership of Anderson Development Corporation. Maxie was a good man that was more involved with the workers than his dad Carl had been. He would soon be asking me to take on some of his new projects.

SCRAPPING A POWER PLANT

MAXIE ANDERSON ASKED ME if I would go to Waco, Texas and scrap the copper wire and the water valves out of the old power plant he had purchased. The plant was built beside the Brazos River, and the water was piped into the power plant. The big, steam-powered motors and generators were gone, but the rest of the infrastructure was intact. Outside of the building were three sets of steel towers; each pair of towers were thirty feet high and sixteen feet apart, with a six-inch by four-inch I-beam sixteen foot long bolted between them. Hanging under the I-Beams were three big transmission wires that ran from the generator building across the yard to the big transformers. The transformers were anchored on concrete pads, and they had small railroad wheels mounted under their frames that transported them from their mountings to the inside of the generator house. Inside the building was a 30-ton crane that could move the heavy loads from one end to the other. The crane operator rode along and was seated in his control booth that was mounted under the crane's frame. Here he could see everything below and control all the crane's movements.

The power plant had thirty-inch piping, with valves that brought the water from the Brazos River into the plant. The steam that was produced would rotate the steam motors, turning the generators and producing electrical power for the town and surrounding areas.

I had to remove the three transmission wires that were hanging thirty feet above. Back in those days, there was no manlift, so after asking everyone if they wanted to climb up there and hearing all the no's, I had to do it myself. I took an oxy acetylene torch with plenty of hose and climbed up each of the towers. I shimmied out on the four-inch-wide beam and cut the hanger bolt that was holding the insulator.

What an amazing ride after the weight of the wire was gone. I bounced up and down for a few minutes before I could continue. I repeated this eight more times until the job was done. After lowering the torch and climbing down, I discovered that sliding along on the beams had worn long slits on both sides of the seat of my pants.

I removed all the valves and adapters and loaded them into barrels, except for the three-foot-diameter valves that rode on the trailer laying down. I hauled all the barrels of valves and adapters to a big pipe yard outside of Houston. The electricity was delivered through town in underground tubes, as each tube had a three-inch lead-covered wire inside. To recover the lead-coated copper wire, we had to get in all the manholes and cut the lead-coated wires. Then we used a come-a-long to pull the lead-coated wire from one maintenance hole to the next. They were cut in four-foot-long pieces and lifted out of the manholes. It took us months to get all the lead-coated copper wire out. We threw the lead-coated wire pieces onto a burn pile that grew about four feet tall and fifteen feet across. I started a fire and melted the lead off. We used homemade rakes to drag through the lead soup, snagging the copper pieces and pulling them out.

As soon as the lead began cooling down and the wires were locked into the lead we were done. After the pile cooled, we started cutting off the copper whiskers that stuck out of the pile of lead. I folded the lead pile over with a forklift, making a lead taco that was now legal in width to haul to Dallas. The copper wire was stuffed in 55-gallon barrels. I took two loaded barrels and weighed them in town on a truck scale to see how much the barrels weighed, then I loaded the copper-filled barrels on a rental truck and hauled them to Dallas to sell them.

I also hauled the giant tacos of melted lead, with all the copper wire pieces sticking out, to a lead manufacturing plant in Dallas. The guys that unloaded my truck at the lead plant had never received a lead taco before, with pieces of copper in it. We continued this process until all the copper and lead was removed. Once we finished, I headed back home to Ambrosia Lake.

Chapter 11

FARMING IN MISSISSIPPI

THE OWNER OF THE trucking company, Maxie, asked me if I would go to Natchez, Mississippi next and set up a farm to feed some cattle he was planning on purchasing. This was going to be another adventure for me, as I would be living in a place that had more bugs and spiders than you could count.

My first challenge was to get a crew together and start preparing the fields. I had seven tractors, some for preparing the ground and some for fertilizing and planting. We had a smaller tractor that had an auger on it to drill holes for the creosote posts we had. One night, we were trying to finish the fencing on the last stretch in the bottom of the levy when the crew got the tractor stuck. One of the men on night shift went to the old farmhouse where I was staying and woke me up, telling me the post hole tractor was stuck, and they could not pull it out.

I ran down to see how bad it was stuck, and as I was headed for the levy, I saw one of the discs unhooked beside the road that should not have been there. I drove over the berm and into the levy; there were tractor lights everywhere. I drove on down past the line of tractors toward the post hole tractor. All the tractors on the farm were stuck in a row at the bottom of the levy. There was nothing that I could do until morning.

After the stores had opened the next day, I purchased a roll of ¾-inch steel cable and cable clamps. I cut the cable in fifteen-feet lengths, and the operators made the tow cables and hooked all the tractors together. I leased a small dozer and built a road down to the bottom side of the levy, close to the front of the post hole tractor. I hooked the dozer up to the post hole tractor and got the operators back in their tractors. When I pulled the first one out, the slack in the cable stretched out and the next tractor came out, and on it went until all the tractors were out of the mud.

Another experience I had I will never forget was discovering what a fish-eating paradise this area was. When I first arrived in Natchez, I was starving when I saw an all-you-can-eat sign. I went into that diner and ordered shrimp. My plate arrived with a big pile of shrimp. I was still trying to clean my plate when the waiter came over and put another platter of shrimp on the table. I learned my lesson about eating at an all-you-can-eat shrimp place in Natchez.

My experience in Mississippi was wonderful. Everybody I worked with was very respectful, and the food was superb.

Chapter 12

RUNNING A SCHOOL BUS COMPANY

MAXIE ANDERSON ASKED ME one day if I would move to Thoreau, New Mexico and take over running the Red Rock Transportation Company, a school bus business that he, my dad, and Carl Lytle had purchased. This time I was not going to be working over the summer months and coming home after the work was done. Maxie was giving me an opportunity to run this business, so I agreed to do it. Thoreau became my new home, and I made a lot of new friends, one of them being Judy Barton.

Neither of us knew it yet, but in a few more years, we would be getting married. However, at that time, I was going to be living in a new world where I was the one responsible for giving directions to others and making things work. The school bus company had 120 buses, twenty of them were spares. Bringing all the kids to school who lived on the Navajo reservation made our buses travel the most dirt road miles any bus company anywhere had traveled.

We supported more than a dozen state run schools with three bus barns: one in Kirkland, one in Gallup, and the main bus barn in Thoreau. All three had fenced-in yards big enough to park and make repairs on all the buses. We had ten mechanics, three of the mechanics drove company service trucks, living in their own areas and were responsible for the buses at those schools. The rest of the mechanics worked in the bus barns. Many of these buses were running over a hundred miles a day. We were unable to find somebody living way out on the Navajo reservation that wanted to drive a school bus. We had to hire a bus driver living somewhere else that drove more miles to pick up the kids and bring them to school and take them home in the evening.

When you are running a school bus business, everybody (secretaries, mechanics, and bosses) are trained and licensed to drive a bus. When you have kids that must get to school or get home, regardless of a problem with a bus or driver, you must have people available to jump in a spare bus and make the run. We worked year-round, making small repairs to keep the buses running, and only had the summer months to do the time-consuming major repairs. Breaking the side windows and cutting up the seats were some of the unnecessary damages that unruly kids were doing all year long to the buses. When this happens, you need to repair the bus ASAP to avoid injuries to the children.

All school buses in New Mexico are given a safety inspection twice a year, conducted by the state police during the school year and before the next school year starts. To keep the school buses in compliance and pass the inspections, it cost the school bus business an average of $30,000 a year above the normal maintenance costs just to replace all the broken windows and the cut-up seat covers. This unnecessary expense was the fault of the school administrations that refused to correct these destructive kids but forced the bus company to suffer the consequences. Some of the kids in school were uncontrollable, and with the lack of support every year from the school districts, the two counties and state, we had to sell the buses and get out of the business in 1979.

Before we sold the business, on the first bad winter storm of 1978, we woke up to two feet of snow, and it slowly melted and rutted the dirt roads for weeks in McKinley County. At 5:00 a.m., the morning after the storm, I called the person in charge of the School Busses at Central Office, informing them of the very deep snow north of Thoreau and I wanted to cancel School in Thoreau and Smith Lake. They did not believe me about the amount of snow that fell that night and decided to have a normal school day. By 7:30 in the morning, many of the school buses were stuck in the bar ditches, along with many private vehicles. Central Office should have canceled school until the county removed the snow before the schools opened.

On that morning, we had thirteen buses stuck; some already had students on board. The bus company's old army wrecker and the three (four-wheel-drive) service trucks worked late that night getting the buses and the private vehicles that were stuck on the roads pulled out. There was one bus left for all of us to tackle the next day. The next morning, we went after that last bus. The driver was a hundred yards from the bridge when the bus slid into the bar ditch. The bus was still trying to move and, with a determined driver who did hundreds of pull forward and back-up maneuvers, the bus ended up in the bottom of the deep arroyo that the bridge crossed over. The bus could have been driven under the bridge if the driver had not stopped.

We used the service trucks to anchor the old wrecker while it winched the bus out of the ditch. Central Office bugged me for days to start running those buses again, but without some major road repairs, the buses would get torn up. I have three picture albums of the damaged roads here at home that I had to show Central Office before the roads were bladed.

WILD BUS STORIES, SOME WITH BAD KIDS, AND REASONS TO FIRE PEOPLE.

On a normal school day, while things were going well again, school was out, and I was headed home when the boss of our Gallup bus yard called me and told me there were kids on a bus in the middle of Gallup, throwing the bottom seats out of the bus windows onto the road. The bus driver had to pull over and turn on her bus lights to prevent an accident. The schools, as usual, did nothing to punish the students.

One time, a night-run bus was stolen from the driver's home, and the thieves were drinking beer and having an enjoyable time when they turned the bus over on a reservation road.

Another bus driver, who was also a teacher at the school, was disciplined by his principal and left the school mad in the middle of the day. He got in his bus and drove ten miles from the school, down a dirt road, and missed the turn-off to his home. He drove the bus off the road and into a pasture before driving over a ditch that was twelve feet deep and twenty feet across. This brand-new bus was going fast when it crashed, smashing into the opposite bank. The front of the bus slid down the vertical bank of the ditch to the bottom, leaving the back of the bus high in the air. The bus body moved forward two feet and made a big crease in the floor of the bus.

The principal called me after he found out about the wreck. That new bus went back to the manufacturer for repairs, and eighteen months later, the manufacturer returned the bus in good condition.

Another incident happened where the principal of another school, who was responsible for locking up the key to our school bus gas tank, was caught by the bus mechanic filling up his own car.

Another wild bus story happened after Christmas break. It was the last day before school started when one of my bus drivers called and told me her bus would not start. I headed out to help her, and seventy-five miles later, I got to the bus, opened the hood, and checked the engine and fan belts. Seeing nothing out of place, I checked the oil and coolant and tried to start the bus. One click from the starter solenoid told me the battery was dead.

I connected my jumper cables and waited a few minutes before trying to start it again. The motor came to life, and I unhooked the cables. I checked the charging system with my voltmeter, and everything was good. Why did the battery die? I walked back to the front of the bus that was parked five feet from the Navajo hogan, facing a window, there they were, some wires rolled up and hanging on a long nail under the window frame.

I looked closely and saw two small pinch clamps that opened wide enough to bite onto the bus's battery posts. Mystery solved: the people living there had wired this hogan with 12v lights they used at night. The bus would have to be started and idle for a while to insure that it would start to make its bus run. Gas was not a problem for them, because it was not theirs, and the bus gas tank was too big for it run out of gas idling for fifteen minutes every night. They must have forgotten to go out and start the bus.

Another bus driver living way out on the reservation called me and said that her bus would not start either. This time, after doing all the checks and trying to start the bus, I realized the battery was also dead. After boosting the battery and trying to start it, I immediately smelled gas. I jumped up on the front bumper and found the gas line had been unscrewed from the carburetor and bent back so a hose could be pushed over the tubing to pump all the gas they could, turning the starter until the battery gave out.

This time, it was not fixable without going back and getting a new gas line. Now all the kids that rode that bus were late to school or did not go that day because the spare bus we drove out to do the run with was late starting the run. Another very selfish stunt that bad people do with no care in the world about the problems they cause; they did not get much gas this way before the battery died anyway.

The best bus story of all time happened after school was over. It took three or four days to get all the buses to the bus barns. Now that school was out, the drivers have their kids at home, and some of them couldn't find a relative or friend to follow them to the bus yard and take them back home. I was still missing one bus, and I was planning to take a mechanic with me after lunch to get the bus when the bus driver came driving through the gate. She parked her bus where we asked her to and came into the office with the keys. She was a good person, and we never had any problems with her.

It was about three weeks later when her bus was brought in for service that the mechanic hollered across the shop at me to come over. He said I should go inside. Wow! What is this? I walked down the aisle to the back of the bus and saw there were hundreds of sheep pills everywhere. She needed to move her sheep herd from one place to another, so she used her sheep-hauling bus. How did she get a sheep to climb up the stairs? Well, nothing was hurt, and this repair was just a high-pressure wash. I still see her around these days, and she is a special friend.

Chapter 13

BECOMING AN OWNER OPERATOR

AFTER THE SCHOOL BUS business was sold, my parents and I bought a new truck and belly dump trailer to haul the uranium ore for United Nuclear. The uranium ore I was hauling came from St. Anthony mine, one hundred miles from the mill. I loaded all the leased trucks and my truck and hauled the uranium ore to Church Rock to the United Nuclear mill. I was doing all repairs, like fixing flat tires, after getting home at night. These were long days, but I was starting to feel like I could finally improve this trucking lifestyle.

I was arriving at Church Rock with my first load of the day on July 16, 1979. I turned and drove through the big gate and up to the scales, when the guard waved and stopped me. He said the tailings dam had cracked and was spilling radioactive water into the Puerco River; the mill was stopping all ore deliveries. I was told to go home after dumping the ore, and the trucking superintendent would call me later.

The radioactive water was a biproduct in the milling of uranium ore, and all the mills had to deal with it. Monitoring the ponds that contained the radioactive water was a top priority. They had a crew that worked day and night monitoring the tailings ponds and berms, as well as the fenced perimeter around them. Unfortunately, this spill would end the uranium mining industry in this area.

I was still hauling uranium ore when Judy and I were married in 1981. Jeremy would also become an adopted son and become a loving part of our family. We lived in my trailer house on an acre of land I purchased beside the bus yard I used to run and were both still adjusting to my early hours. I was leaving at 3:30 in the morning, hauling two loads of uranium ore from St. Anthony to Church Rock every day and getting back home at 10:30 at night. It was around two a.m. one morning when we were suddenly woken by a loud crashing noise. We both jumped out of bed, and I turned the lamp on, and we saw one of our horses pulling his head out of the window and backing away from the trailer. He left the curtains he was trying to nibble on hanging out of the window opening. Well, keeping the gate shut to the corrals and repairing the screen was a priority for me now.

My time as an owner operator span many years, hauling uranium, coal, sand, gravel, cattle, buildings, heavy equipment, alfalfa hay, and the water for the rodeo arena at the bi-county fair every year, as well as the sawdust for the show animals and show barn. I even dug up some big pinon trees in Ambrosia Lake and hauled them to the fairgrounds.

I got a job with Quivera Mining Corporation as a mechanic at the old Kerr-McGee mill and I did my farm work every evening and the trucking on the weekends This new job would provide my family with insurance that covered Lawrence and a steady paycheck.

Chapter 14

A CHALLENGING BIRTH

THE DAY THAT CHANGED OUR LIVES

MAN, I AM TIRED, but just one more flat tire to fix. I look at my watch and see it is 2:30 in the morning; I have been fixing flats for four hours. I need to get the truck ready to go and not have any problems when I head out to St. Anthony tomorrow to load the other trucks, and mine as well, with uranium ore. I sure hope dad does not have any trouble loading all the trucks today, since I am taking the day off.

It seems like forever since I got to the hospital, and I am tired from not sleeping last night. I have sat here and read every poster in this room a dozen times, and I still cannot remember what they say. The nurses at the desk have been talking and laughing about something, but who knows what it is. One of them asked me if I would like a cup of coffee, and I needed one for sure, since I have not eaten anything this morning. The quiet of the waiting area is disturbed by a nurse rushing through the big doors and running up to the girls at the desk, asking them where the oxygen cart is. The three of them run out, and I just sit there, wondering to myself what this is about. A few minutes later, the nurse came running through the waiting room with the cart and through the double doors. I ask the nurses standing by the desk what happened, and they tell me they need the oxygen in the delivery room.

A big knot forms in my throat because I am waiting for my wife Judy to have a C-Section and deliver our son this morning.

On this day me, Judy and Lawrence's big brother Jeremy, begin a journey of never-ending challenges, but with lots of prayers along the way, that would change our lives forever. We learned that we had to keep moving forward and trust in the Lord, regardless of the difficulties, and to never, never give up. This was the beginning of our story living with cerebral palsy.

Judy became pregnant with our first child and her due date was getting close. Our plan was to go back to Gallup to the same doctor that had delivered Jeremy to have a scheduled C-section. We had paid for the hospital delivery and the doctor in advance because we did not have insurance. Judy's doctor set the date, and everything was going to plan. Once Judy was admitted, she would stay all night and have the scheduled C-section the next morning.

Judy and I were unaware of any problems until the nurse came to Judy's room and told us, that while Lawrence was being examined by the doctor, he had a seizure and was being prepped for a flight to BCMC (Bernalillo County Medical Center) in Albuquerque, New Mexico. Judy never saw or talked to her doctor after leaving the delivery room from his birth till now almost forty-one years later. Well, things were in God's hands now.

Judy had to stay in the hospital to recover from the C-section, so I drove to Albuquerque (one hundred and twenty miles away). I was there waiting outside the emergency room when the medics arrived with Lawrence. He was placed in the regular ICU because the pediatric ICU was full; I was allowed to stay in the ICU with him. His little hands, arms, and feet had been poked everywhere to get an IV in. I sat there, holding his hand and praying for hours and hours and three days later he finally had a bowel movement, which he hadn't proven to do yet, now they would release him, and our family could finally be together at home.

After we all got out of the hospitals and were home, we started focusing on our new lifestyle. We were told that he was delivered three weeks early, and sometimes babies will be born that can't respond to lights and sounds right away, and that happens now and then. Well, if everything was done correctly, why was the nurse running around hunting for the oxygen cart? I had a feeling inside of me that said the oxygen cart should have been in the delivery room for this type of incident. I regret not being in the room with Judy and seeing what happened.

It makes me wonder why her doctor would not see her and has never talked to her since. I thought when a doctor does surgery on a patient, he would check on them and see how they were doing, but not her doctor; he did not care. Lawrence is going to live with these challenges for the rest of his life. Fortunately for Lawrence, and us, Jesus is going to be with us from now into eternity.

Chapter 15

LOVING AND LIVING WITH CEREBRAL PALSY

WE ALL HAVE PERFECT expectations of a newborn child when we are waiting for their birth. And for most births, it is a wondrously blessed day. But for the unfortunate child with complications, there are also severe challenges that are a part of the birth as well. When this happens to some couples, a single mom, or an entire family, they could be thrown into a state of mind that starts to question everything they had ever planned. How are we going to continue making decisions by ourselves? Who is going to listen to you in your time of desperation? When a baby is born with any challenges, mentally or physically, there is only one person you can rely on, and that person is Jesus.

In many cases, a young couple is coerced into believing the professionals with their personal opinions about how you should manage these challenges, or it might be family members or relatives that make suggestions. Although meaning well, it can sometimes hurt your feelings and make matters worse. It wasn't any different with us; we had our share of opinions and criticisms about Lawrence. Not only are the lives of the parents being changed, but the concerns of the siblings, family members, relatives, and friends are with the child that they cannot help.

Lawrence's challenges in life would be a learning experience for everyone. Fortunately for our son, with Jesus watching over us, it came down to one four-letter word: LOVE.

Brother George Brittain was pastor of First Baptist Church in Thoreau, and he and his wife Flois were always blessing us with prayers of encouragement and support. They understood that Judy and I were blessed to be given an angel to raise. Pastor George and Flois treated us like we were their kids. Every Sunday, Flois would walk up to me, give me a kiss on the cheek, and straighten my collar. She was the one in charge. After Brother George retired, his son, Brother Bob Brittain, moved back to Grants and became pastor of First Baptist in Thoreau. He and his wife Judy have always been there for us; we love them dearly.

Lawrence was diagnosed with cerebral palsy after his birth. This condition slowed down his reaction time to everyday events. It takes him much more time to process what he sees or feels. When Lawrence was young, we thought, at times, he did not hear us or see the light turn on, but after a while, he would respond.

Lawrence's doctor wanted him to see a neurologist, so we went to BCMC in Albuquerque for the checkup. The doctor took about two minutes, standing out in the hallway, with Lawrence cradled in his arm. He spun around in a circle 360 degrees in both directions, watching his eyes and then told us we should think about giving him up to the state. His brief diagnosis of Lawrence was he was blind or brain blind, (not able to compute what his eyes were seeing). The doctor felt Lawrence would be too much of a burden for us to raise him. Well, he did not know my wife and I very well.

We were upset, hurt, and wanted to get away from that fool as fast as we could, stunned by his diagnosis and his professional opinion that we could not talk about it for a while. There was no way that our son did not deserve to live on this earth like everyone else. I was thinking to myself, how many couples would consider this guy's advice? Fortunately for Lawrence, he has a family that never gives up.

After paying an enormous bill for that ridiculous diagnosis, we headed back home to continue our lives without the stupidity of a bunch of overpaid professionals. Lawrence was slowly starting to improve, and he would prove that neurologist wrong.

After we had finally survived all of Lawrences first few months of hospital visits in Albuquerque and were settling down, we started learning to live with cerebral palsy, seizures, seizure meds, scoliosis, chronic constipation, and many sleepless nights with Lawrence. Judy and I, with Jeremy's help (Lawrence's big brother), were there for Lawrence every day and night, giving him all the love and nurturing that we could give. Lawrence, despite having such challenges and with all our prayers, refused to quit on us either.

Judy has been the person that has given all her time for Lawrence's well-being all these years. She has been by his side for every moan or cry that he might utter day or night. She gets up three or more times a night to check on him, seeing if he needs to be repositioned and to stretch his legs or help him get his arms under the covers.

If it weren't for Judy and all her sacrifices, we could not have survived caring for Lawrence. She has been taking care of Lawrence while living this 24-hour-a-day life for forty years now, changing three diapers a day, making all the special meals and drinks, and making sure he is sitting in the right position for every meal. No human being has ever given more for the love of a child than she has.

As several months passed, we noticed Lawrence was starting to react more when he heard our voices. He would turn his eyes toward us much faster as we spoke, and he was starting to react more by looking toward the light when it was turned on or off.

This was the time in our lives when I had to transition from working for the Quivera uranium mill, to working for the Santa Fe Coal Company. I would be gone fourteen hours a day for two sets of four days on and four days off, and then do two sets of four nights on and four days off. This would be a huge burden on Judy while I was gone those days.

After a few months had passed, Lawrence started to army crawl around the living room and trying to sit up. He was seeing things more clearly, even with nystagmus in his eyes (a rapid, uncontrolled jerking of the eyes that I believe is caused from cerebral palsy in some situations). Among all his toys, Lawrence had a bunch of square-headed throw toys that were his favorites. These toys would make talking noises when he threw them at us to catch, and it really made him laugh when we missed catching them and they fell to the floor. This game was his favorite game, and everybody that came to visit had to play it with him. When we took Lawrence to the ranch, he got excited to see and pet the horses, and he really liked riding on Peewee around the yard. Peewee was a Shetland pony that was very gentle with him.

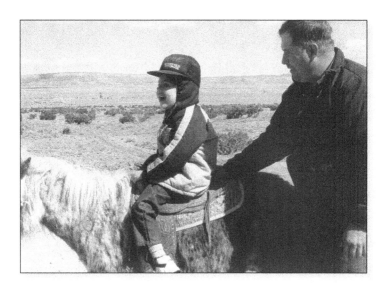

Lawrence riding Peewee at the ranch with uranium mines in the background

During this breakthrough period, he started smiling more and playing with us. However, it was in this stage of growth that his scoliosis in his back was becoming more severe.

Lawernce's doctor suggested that the best cure for his scoliosis would be surgery to pin his back, but we were too afraid of what might happen to someone so fragile. We knew that fusing or putting pins in his back would mean locking his back in a straight position. We had to weigh the risks that he would have to take.

1. He might not survive the surgery.
2. He might be paralyzed.
3. He might become harder to feed.
4. He might be locked in a position and would not be able to reach and get things.
5. He might be limited to the amount of time he could stay in his wheelchair before getting pressure sores.

We decided, in the end, to decline the doctor's advice.

We did not have any insurance when Lawrence was born, and all the professionals and specialists that we met and worked with never told us Lawrence was eligible for Medicaid. All the bills were ours until he turned sixteen, except for the folding wheelchair that was given to Lawrence from the Elks Club. One of their members that we did not know, with a big heart, heard about Lawrence and blessed us with the wheelchair. This was his first wheelchair that we used for many years.

We were told about the DD Waiver program in New Mexico when Lawrence was four years old, but it took Lawrence twelve years to be enrolled because the waiting list was so long. With no help coming for Lawrence, it would be our own ingenuity to build what we needed. We became the most proactive parents Lawrence could have. From that day forward, we would do whatever it took to make Lawrence's life as comfortable as we could.

This is a list of the things we built for our son:

1. Corrective back brace for scoliosis
2. Wrist braces
3. Ankle braces
4. Stander-walker
5. Wheelchair that lifts him up off the floor and moves him around the house
6. Wheelchair lift for our first used van
7. Building 50 feet of steel wheelchair ramp for the house
8. Remodeled his bathroom and installed a small jacuzzi tub
9. Different types of motivational tools
10. Recliner-style leg rest for both of his wheelchairs
11. Wheelchair lift on motorhome
12. Installed identical rails in motorhome bathroom that are in the house
13. Built a sucker machine to vacuum and clean his mouth and throat

Chapter 16

SEIZURES, NEUROLOGISTS, AND MEDICATION

ONE DAY, LAWRENCE HAD his first grand mal seizure. It started with a groan and then a frozen face and stiff arms and legs. His body would jerk and contort, and you could see that his breathing was restricted for periods of time before he started breathing again. This was repeated several times while the seizure was going on.

During the seizure, we all jumped in the car and headed for the emergency room in Grants. The seizure stayed strong while we were driving for fifteen minutes, then it started to weaken. After thirty minutes driving, we arrived at the emergency room and the seizure had stopped, leaving Lawrence very sleepy and exhausted, and the rest of us scared from witnessing the seizure. Once in the emergency room, we described the seizure to the doctor, and he prescribed Lawrence with his first seizure med. This med would be his first line of defense against seizures, but not his last.

Lawrence was now six years old, and he was starting to have seizures on a regular basis. Seizures, unfortunately, are a part of the lives of some children with cerebral palsy. Throughout our son's life, he has had the grand mal, and the lesser and more frequent startle-type seizures. The lesser startle-type events are more like he felt something funny. He becomes startled and moves his head and arms and legs for a few seconds. It is usually over in a few moments, but it still leaves him tired for a while.

Lawrence has been with different neurologists all his life. Every time he got a different one, they would always decide that there was a different seizure med that would slow down the seizures. The first med that was prescribed by the doctor in the emergency room was bad for his teeth, which we finally learned about the problem from his first neurologist. He changed the medication, and we had to wait three months to see his improvements. He has had many neurologists move away over the years, so every time a different neurologist diagnoses him, he changes his meds.

After this cycle of different neurologists, changing meds, and no improvement, Judy and I finally figured out what the problem was. It took Lawrence more than three months to get used to a med, and it was always three months between his appointments. We told the next neurologist to leave his meds alone and give him more time to get used to it. Well, that was the problem; he started having less of the startle and grand mal seizures and was more awake and able to play again due to the meds.

Documenting the seizures was necessary to see if Lawrence was getting better or worse. Judy has kept a seizure logbook for many years, and she can tell if he is having a problem. His last neurologist was excited to see the actual time and duration of the seizures that were recorded for years, telling us she was going to try to get her other patients to start keeping a logbook as well.

Chapter 17

BACK, ARM, AND ANKLE BRACES

LAWRENCE HAD VERY WEAK muscle tone that was attributed to CP because he could not move and exercise like a normal child, but after many years, we believe the seizure meds have contributed to it also, making him so drowsy. As his scoliosis became more evident, I decided to build Lawrence a corrective back brace. I bought six feet of the largest diameter PVC pipe I could find and cut off a piece that was long enough, and then I cut it longways.

I took a small propane burner and warmed it up enough to flatten the pipe like a sheet of paper, spraying it with cool water to harden it and keep it flat. I measured our son in several places, all the way around from under his arms to his waist. I started forming the brace, allowing enough space for a lining, which was glued to the inside. It took a while to form it, working small areas of the sheet at a time, warming it up and cooling it down. Once I had it close to the correct size, it became more time-consuming because it had to fit without any pinch points. I hinged it in the back vertically so we could place it around Lawrence easily. I cut a six-inch hole in the back that aligned with the bulge of the scoliosis and glued the foam lining inside the brace for comfort.

When he had it on, there was a two-inch-wide gap from top to bottom in the front, which I fastened with shoelaces, crisscrossing from bottom to top; this made it adjustable as he grew. I covered it with sturdy fabric and made a big pocket over the hole on the back, where a foam ball was inserted to put pressure on the bulge of the scoliosis and help slow it down. A firmer ball would be put in to increase the pressure.

Lawrence would only wear it for short periods at a time. Our hope was to slow the scoliosis and keep it manageable as he grew. Our son's wrists and ankles had little muscle tone as well. His wrists would flatten and his ankles would turn sideways when he tried to crawl on the carpet and stand in his walker. I made him wrist and ankle braces to give him the support he needed, which led to him army crawling and standing in his walker. As soon as he was in the stander, he was much more aware of his surroundings and would throw and watch the toys as they were thrown. We try to keep him in the stander until he got tired; the time he spent standing increased as his muscles grew stronger.

Chapter 18

POTTY CHAIR AND FOAMS

LAWRENCE HAS HAD CHRONIC constipation all his life and with his scoliosis, sitting on a potty chair is difficult. They do not make a toilet seat or a potty chair that helps a child with severe scoliosis (ninety degrees in Lawrence's case). When Lawrence was seated on his new potty chair for the first time, he sat there folded over the armrest. To improve the seating, and make it more comfortable for him, I took four squares of one-inch-thick by sixteen-inch by sixteen-inch foam pads and cut a six-inch round hole in the middle of them. I stacked four of the pads on top of each other, making a soft seat that helps him sit upright by allowing his lower hip to sink in deeper into the foams.

We used the potty chair seatbelt around his waist and mounted a gait belt a few inches higher on the chair at his chest to give him added support, while sitting safely in the chair; this made it more comfortable and safer for him. Judy takes the opportunity to shave his face and brush his teeth while he is in his chair. When brushing his teeth, we use the sucker machine to suck out his throat and around his gums and teeth. He has been using his modified chair for twenty years and it seems to still be working.

Chapter 19

EATING, DRINKING, AND CHOKING

LAWRENCE IS A GOOD eater and eats the same food that we do. Judy and I chop his food into small pieces so he will not choke. It takes him a little longer to chew and sip his drink, but he swallows safely. When he is eating and drinking, he sits in a set position in his wheelchair to keep his body in the best position for swallowing. If he gets tired of waiting and wants a drink or a bite, he will lean over in his wheelchair and reach for his choice. He must drink liquids all day to keep hydrated.

When he was younger, he would get some M&Ms for a snack. He liked them so much, he started grabbing them himself and putting them in his mouth. This treat was bad for his teeth, but they helped him start eating on his own. Choking is a problem for Lawrence when eating, drinking, and especially when taking meds. We must be careful about it.

When Lawrence was thirty-five, we had laid him down for his nap fifteen minutes after taking his meds. While he was reclining in his chair, he coughed up the meds into his throat, and then he gasped for a breath of air, breathing the mixture into his lungs. I lifted him out of the chair and placed him on his stomach on my lap, trying to get him to spit it out. Without any success Judy, Lawrence and I jumped in the car and rushed him forty miles to the hospital in Grants. Once in the emergency room, we explained to the nurse what had happened. The doctor came in to examine him and became very skeptical of our story. After his examination, the doctor told us that he did not think Lawrence had inhaled something; his opinion was he had pneumonia. He told us that people that are confined to wheelchairs are more likely to have pneumonia because of their lack of mobility, and Lawrence was acting the same way as them.

We had to get him admitted, and Judy would have to stay with him. I rushed back home and got all his meds, Judy's meds, and their extra clothes and came back to the hospital. Once I brought Lawrence' meds in the room, the nurse said she had to give them to their pharmacist so they could control administering the correct doses. That was not going to work, because Judy takes extra time letting Lawrence get ready for each of his meds. Lawrence knows when he is ready for his meds, and it is a slow process. He will open his mouth to take the med on his own. If he is hurried, he will start coughing, gasping for air, and then he will start choking. He might have to wait up to thirty minutes before he can continue.

Finally, the staff understood and left us alone with his meds. Judy had learned the secret it takes to administer Lawrence's meds for thirty years at that point.

When his hospital stay was over, and we were leaving his room, the doctor told us that we were right; Lawrence did not have pneumonia. He was discharged after three days. I asked the nurse if I could keep the suction bowl and the tubing that we had used during his stay. She told me she would have to ask her boss about it and, after five minutes, she came running out to us in the parking lot with a new suction assembly and gave it to me.

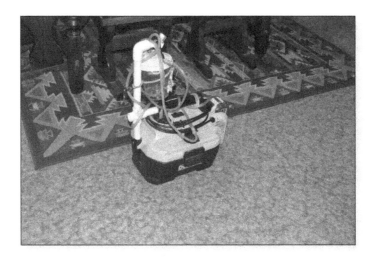

Sucker machine I designed after Lawrences choking incident

During the entire encounter, we became good friends with the hospital staff, and they went out of their way to help us. After getting home, I made a sucker machine that night, using the assembly they gave us and my shop vac. I wanted to be ready if we had to suck out his throat again. The next morning, I ordered several sets of the vacuum collection kits and two smaller 120 volt or battery-powered shop vacs, which provide a strong vacuum. I mounted a stand arm on both machines to carry the collection jar and wrap the hose and nozzle around it. I clean it after each use and keep a charged battery on it that would last four days before changing it out. One machine is the spare since a failure could take a week to replace it. We still use it for cleaning out his mouth after brushing his teeth in the mornings and evenings. We always take it with us wherever we go.

Chapter 2 0

SLEEPING

AFTER LUNCH, SUPPER, AND taking his meds, Lawrence sits up for at least one hour before taking his nap or going to bed. The hour long waits ensure that Lawrence digested the food and meds before laying down. He sleeps on a queen-size select comfort bed that we keep soft and comfortable, placed on the floor without its base. We placed cloth-covered beanbags against his bed to soften the fall if he rolled off his bed. If Lawrence happened to roll in front of his door, we could not open it without hurting him. I re-mounted the door to swing outward instead of inward.

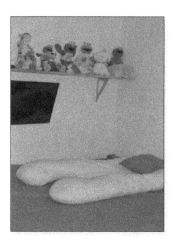

Lawrences bed with his TV and body pillow

He has his own wall-mounted TV above his bed, close enough where he can watch videos. He only makes it about ten minutes before falling asleep. He has his own portable radiator heater with a thermostat that keeps his bedroom at a constant temperature. We purchased a body pillow for sleeping that keeps him on his back or side and prevents him from rolling off the bed. Later, the beanbags were removed, and his bed was put back on the base. No more strained backs for Judy and I when he goes to bed or when we change him. We keep monitors in his room that alert us in case he makes a noise and needs help. Judy has checked on him three or four times every night for his lifetime.

Chapter 21

BATHING AND SHOWERING

WHEN LAWRENCE STARTED GAINING weight, it became a challenge for Judy and me to bathe him. We first used a shower chair that we pushed into the shower. The shower stall had a four-inch rise on the floor that had to be overcome by lifting him and the chair over it. Once in the stall, one of us had to hold him in the chair and keep him from leaning over. When his shower was over, we banged and bounced our way out of the shower. What a challenge that was.

As part of the DD Waiver, we received some home improvement money that we used to get a battery-powered lift that was hanging from a trolley and moved along rails that were mounted to the ceiling. The rails went from his bedroom to his shower in his bathroom. Wow, what an improvement this was over the shower chair, but after his shower, he would be freezing by the time we got him lowered onto his bed.

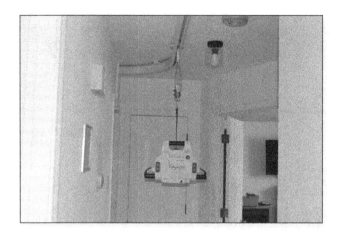

Barrier-Free lift that raises Lawrence up and moves him into his bathroom

Our next try after the shower was bathing. The problem that we were dealing with was the tub that they installed was not what we ordered. They installed a walk-in tub in the guest bathroom with a six-foot-long piece of rail above it. This caused me to move the living room lift to the guest bathroom before each bath, getting him ready for the bath in his bedroom, putting him in his wheelchair on a towel, and wheeling him through the house to the guest bathroom where the walk-in tub was. This method was much easier for our son and us, but it came with extra work and many concerns and worries about suspending Lawrence over a tub full of water and having something fail on the lift or the rails and trolley. A failure would drop him in the water, and the tub door that opened inward could not open.

So, Judy and I purchased the jacuzzi style tub we wanted and did our own bathroom makeover in his bathroom that is next to his bedroom. Lawrence gets ready for his bath in his bedroom, he gets put into his bath harness and hooked up to his Voyager lift that lifts him up and carries him along a rail that is mounted to the ceiling and travels from his bed, down the hallway and into his bathroom and lowers him into the bathtub.

Chapter 22

IMPORTANCE OF RE-POSITIONING WITH WHEELCHAIRS

REPOSITIONING AND CHANGING CHAIRS help stop swelling and pressure sores for Lawrence. Even when traveling, being confined in a wheelchair for long hours without repositioning can be painful. Judy and I are guilty of this because when we are driving somewhere, waiting for appointments, and then going some more, it is easy to forget to check and reposition Lawrence. His chair has a formed mold that matches his scoliosis and requires that he be seated correctly in it.

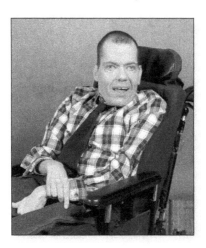

Lawrence in his wheelchair

The problem for people that are confined in their chairs for lengthy periods of time is slipping forward. When Lawrence slips forward, he moves out of the comfortable molded seat and becomes uncomfortable. We must be very aware of this and reposition him in his chair when needed. The best indicator that he has slipped forward is seeing the normal distance of his head from the top of the headrest has changed. Tying people down correctly is also important. Lawrence's wheelchair has pneumatic tires for a softer ride, as solid tires have no give at all, and bumps can make the ride very rough.

Our son gets swollen and cold feet after an hour or two sitting in his chair at home or when we go to town. He has seen doctors and therapists for a couple of years about it, but no solution has been found. Judy decided to put pillows on his footrests to elevate his feet, and the cold and swollen problem went away. I built him an adjustable leg rest like a recliner that fits in the footrest mounting bracket holes on the chair, so I did not have to modify the chair, just remove the factory footrests, and it has eliminated discomfort in Lawrence's legs.

Another problem that happens with people in wheelchairs is while shopping or walking around and enjoying the surroundings they are always in front where they only see strangers. Lawrence's nystagmus (a rapid jerking from side to side of the eye) made it hard for him to focus on anything. Now, one of us walks along beside him, holding his hand and making him feel more comfortable. When we are traveling, his chair is strapped to tiedown brackets I made, because tiedown brackets do not come with a wheelchair anymore. If you do not have the brackets, you must make sure that the chair is secured safely onto the main frame of the chair, so it can withstand the starts and stops of a vehicle.

Another problem with wheelchairs is how the tires move on carpet and linoleum. After many years of turning the wheelchair on carpet or linoleum, the tire that is not moving is spinning around, causing the carpet to start pulling up from the seams and eventually ruining the carpet. The chair will also start damaging linoleum over time from continuous travel and turning in the same spot. To keep this from happening, try to push the wheelchair forward or backward to a different place when turning, if you have available room.

I use pneumatic tires on Lawrence's chair instead of solid tires to soften the ride, but they are more damaging to the carpet or linoleum. Most wheelchairs will come with solid tires, so there is no maintenance required, like having to keep pneumatic tires aired up, but the ride to me is worth the effort.

Chapter 23

ENTERTAINING AND THERAPISTS

WE HAVE BEEN KEEPING our son entertained all his life. He likes to sit beside one of us at his table and play with his toys by throwing them in baskets or playing catch with us. He really likes to fake you out when you miss the catch and then must go pick the toy off the floor. When that happens, he will break out in laughter. He likes playing with his piano and many of his other toys and games.

Our son has been seeing his speech, physical, and occupational therapists for many years. He really enjoys getting to interact with them and all their projects. They all come to our house for an hour on their different days.

John, his physical therapist, has been working with Lawrence for twenty years now and comes once a week. We help John get Lawrence into his stander, with his ankle braces on, and John uses an assortment of toys to keep him entertained while his legs muscles are stretched out to become stronger. He makes Lawrence use his full range of motion in both arms and wrists, keeping his back as straight as he can. John has always helped us when Lawrence is eligible to upgrade his wheelchair. After learning about the accessories that are available for a wheelchair, I have been adding things to make the wheelchair better as well.

Cheryl is Lawrence's speech therapist and has been assisting Lawrence for years. She has explored all the communication devices that are available for him. Because of his challenging vision, she uses a computer with a big touch screen monitor that is helping him see things better. She has downloaded many learning apps and games that he really likes. He has a piano board and several musical instruments he can play with her assistance while she sings along. Many games, like Tic-Tac-Toe and Firefighter, keep him interested. She also got him a portable spray tank that hangs from his wheelchair and it has a spray nozzle he can water his flowers with.

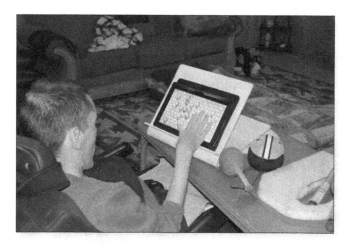

Lawrence playing with his computer

Cheryl has helped Lawrence make his choices with pictures that are laid on an easel and then push his yes and no switches that loudly respond. We let Lawrence have choices in picking which restaurant he wants to eat at by showing him the pictures of the restaurants. He makes his choice by reaching out and touching the restaurant picture he wants. He also picks what he wants to eat with different pictures of his favorite meals from the restaurant he chooses. Lawrence has responded well to Cheryl's ideas.

Melanie is his occupational therapist and does all kinds of art projects with Lawrence that get a little messy, but he enjoys doing them with her. He does fingerpainting, throwing painted objects onto a picture paper, and making his own pictures to give away or hang in his room. Melanie was also using the local swimming pool to enhance his awareness of things around him. He enjoys splashing his friends and pushing the beach ball around while floating in the pool.

Judy and I designed a room for him in our house that has many things he plays with. He has an electric train and a ski lift on a table he starts with a push switch, which he can reach from his wheelchair. He has a bowling alley with an aiming tube I built and several push button-activated animals that move and growl with lit-up scary eyes, as well as lots of throwing games to choose from. He has airplanes flying around in circles overhead that he likes to watch. We always take his favorite toys with us when we travel to keep him entertained.

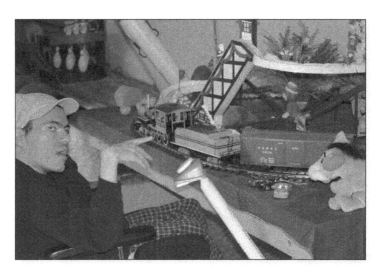

Lawrence playing with his electric train and ski lift

His older brother, Jeremy, returned from the Iraq War and got married and was living in Colorado Springs. For Lawrence to visit his brother, we bought a used motorhome and loaded it up with the devices he needed. We take his wheelchair tray for games and eating. Traveling in this motorhome was exciting for Lawrence. Different noises and feeling the different movements made when turning and slowing down the motorhome kept him awake for hours.

After his brother moved to Yakima, Washington, we bought a new and bigger motorhome. Lawrence can now sit in the front, tied down between us so he can see the big trucks and scenery go by. Going on trips to see his brother has become his favorite thing to do. I installed the same type rails in the bathroom ceiling in the motorhome as in the house, and I mounted a wheelchair lift on the side entrance of the motorhome so he can be loaded safely.

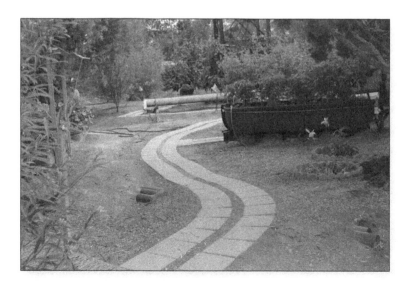

The wheelchair accessible garden we built for Lawrence

I built Lawrence a big garden, with raised plots and walkways through it, where he can wheel up beside them and water the plants. Once the vegetables have ripened, he can reach and pick some vegetables. He also has grapes growing around an arbor he sits under where he can see and pick them and a small orchard he can pick fruit from as well.

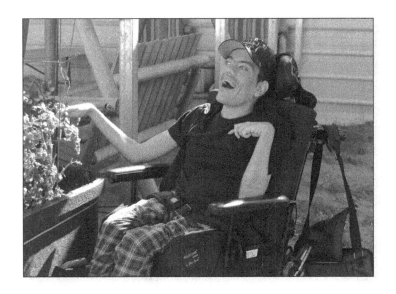

Lawrence is picking green tomatoes

Chapter 24

AED, WHY TAKE A CHANCE?

JUDY AND I HAVE been through many mandatory first-aid classes for many years and have been told how to use the AED and why it is so important as a life-and-death tool in emergencies. The problem that arose during the training classes over many years is if you really did need an AED, where is it? I asked our trainer where the AED was located. We were told that they did not have one because they were too pricy, and if we needed an AED to call 911, or go to the fire station, the library, or to the emergency room. If the cost of the device keeps a business from having one, the person you are trying to save might not survive. Well, I know if we need an AED to save a life in our home or vehicle, those options will not work. We bought our own AED and have it with us and ready whenever we need it.

Chapter 25

WORKING FOR THE COAL MINE

JUDY AND I HAVE always had our forever job of caring for Lawrence, even though I had to keep working to provide for our living. After my employment ended with Quivera Mining Corporation (formerly Kerr-McGee), I was hired as a mechanic for Santa Fe Coal Company. This new job was a blessing from God, but I started out on the wrong foot. My boss at my new job was not happy with me giving Kerr-McGee two weeks' notice. The next day, the maintenance supervisor called and asked when I was planning on being at work. Everybody I talked with during the hiring process knew about my pledge to give my old employer a two-week notice. He told me no one does that anymore, and I needed to get there ASAP. Well, I should have read *How to Get Hired by a Coal Mine for Dummies*. I have worked for some good, understanding people, but my new boss was going to be my greatest challenge. As expected on my first day, I was treated like the mine had been shut down until I got there. After my training period, riding along in the fuel and lube trucks, I was sent out on my own.

My boss's problem with me was my experience working on heavy equipment. Rather than accept that I might know something, he just sent me out on the fuel or lube trucks. For the next years, the equipment operators would tell me he came by to see if I had performed all the maintenance on their machine. I felt like he was trying to find a reason to get rid of me.

Things were getting so bad that Judy had encouraged me to quit. Several of the men on the crew had asked him what was going on, and a few of them went over his head, to the maintenance superintendent, but nothing seemed to help. But with Jesus's help, I stayed the course and was able to endure all the stress. Judy would ask me why I was still putting up with all of this, but we both knew the answer. We needed this job financially and for the insurance.

After a few more months, the maintenance superintendent finally stirred up the foremen, and my boss was transferred to another department. With a different foreman, things started improving for me. I finally advanced from tech one pay scale to tech three in a couple of months. He put the next new hire on the fuel and lube rotation like it was meant to be. This gave a new hire an opportunity to learn the layout of the mine and the different types of equipment while servicing them.

Now I was working on all the equipment, sometimes training new mechanics that were learning to do the repairs. I was slowly advancing and starting to fill in for the boss's absence. Now the stress I had delt with for years was gone.

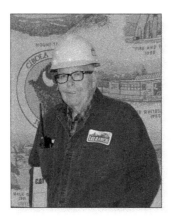

Foreman at the coal mine

With things going well at work, it was Judy's transportation problems that started to fester. Judy drove the old van to town until it died one day and would not start. She had Lawrence with her and was upset and angry, trying to decide what to do. She sat there in the parking lot, unaware that the wait time had given the vapor locked fuel system time to cool down. Finally, she tried to start it again, and the old van fired up and got them home. As soon as I got home from work, I was informed about their experience. We both knew we had to buy a more reliable vehicle.

While I worked for the coal mine, we financed a Transit Connect van with a new wheelchair lift in it. No more lifting and straining our backs, and Lawrence would stay seated comfortably in his wheelchair. This vehicle became our best investment for Lawrence. Now Judy could load and unload Lawrence by herself and was able to easily tie his wheelchair down and do what she needed to do. We would now be able to have a dependable and comfortable ride for Lawrence wherever we went, even on those long trips towing it behind the motorhome.

Chapter 26

INTERESTING STORIES

THE WELDERS WERE MAKING repairs on the bed of a two-hundred-and-forty-ton haul truck in the coal mine shop and needed some two-inch pipe. Two of the welders ran down to the boneyard looking for a piece. They found a straight piece that was long enough and leaned over to pick it up. One grabbed the pipe around the outside, and the other stuck his fingers inside the pipe. As they raised the pipe up, a mouse bit one of the guys' fingers sticking inside. With a holler, he dropped the pipe and came back to the shop. His finger was cleaned up and bandaged. The safety man had to be called and when he arrived and looked at it, he sent the guy to town for a tetanus shot and the rest of the day off. This incident would become a safety topic for our company for a while.

One of the men on the crew went into the break room for lunch. He warmed up his meal and started eating. He got up after a few minutes and left the room. We all finished our lunch and headed back to work, but the guy never came back. What happened to the guy that did not finish his lunch? He had forgotten to put his denture adhesive on and was unable to eat. He went to his toolbox and used some automotive silicone on his teeth. As soon as he placed his teeth in his mouth, he began throwing up and became nauseous. He was washing his mouth out for hours to get the silicone smell and taste out of his mouth. No safety topic this time; the guy was too embarrassed to tell anyone what he had done for months.

The shovel operator's job required him to check the lube tanks and inform maintenance if they needed to be topped off. The maintenance foreman and a couple of mechanics would go to the shovel on night shift and do a walk-around on the shovel; the mechanics brought the lube trailer with them to do that. On many occasions, when the mechanics arrived back at the shop, they noticed they forgot to lock the hitch and the lube trailer was missing. They always tried to hurry back, find the lube buggy and bring it back to the shop before someone else found out. Unfortunately, when a truck driver or the production boss found it, they would call maintenance and ask them if that was the new parking place for the lube buggy.

Chapter 27

WHAT HAPPENED TO JEREMY?

OUR OLDEST SON JEREMY, who was Lawrence's protector while they were both at school, has been the most loving brother anyone could ever want. He was always helping Lawrence when they were together. Jeremy had started going to church here at First Baptist in Thoreau in his early teens. He has always loved Jesus and has been witnessing for the Lord all his life. After he graduated from high school, he was always involved with the youth groups here in Thoreau and with the groups in Grants. He volunteered to go on a mission and was selected to go to a small town in Washington to help minister and witness to a small church in Chehalis, Washington.

After he finally came back home, he decided to go to school in Oklahoma City. It was there at a church in Arcadia, Oklahoma, where he was the youth pastor, that he met a young lady from another church that really impressed him. They both went on a mission trip to Panama, with Jeremy being the medic and Adela, the young lady, was the pharmacist. After this mission trip ended and, after building up his courage, he finally asked her out on a date.

Well, as their relationship was developing, Jeremy decided to join the army; Adela and Jeremy were married that same year. Jeremy was an army medic and served in Iraq. While he was headed to Bagdad in convoy, the Humvee, he was in wrecked and hurt some discs in his neck and back. While there, he had to sleep sitting in a chair to help with the pain.

Adela was an only child, from Timisoara, Romania, and she lived through the evil, socialist-run government oppression at that time. She learned to speak English so she could interpret for the missionaries that would come occasionally to Romania. It was in Timisoara where a big revival happened, and Luis Palau was there. This is where she accepted Jesus as her personal Lord and Savior and fell in love with His Word. She would dream of getting out of her country and going to live in America and, someday, finding someone else that loved Jesus the way she did and get married. She eventually met a missionary that would bring her back here to America. She got a pharmacist degree from University of Oklahoma by working jobs and not wasting money playing, like most of the kids. During her time in pharmacy school in Oklahoma is where she met Jeremy.

Now they live in Salem, Oregon and have given us three wonderful grandchildren: Lucas, Sammy, and Emma. Jeremy is a physician assistant and Adela is a pharmacist, who currently works part-time as the women's ministry director at their local church.

FIGHTING OFF DIABETES

WELL, AFTER WORKING ALL my life doing different jobs, that kept me away from home made eating fast food the only answer for me. I was not aware of the damage I was doing to my health by eating all those carbohydrates for years. I have learned, as I have grown older that my A1C was slowly rising. (A1C is the standard for measuring blood sugar management in people with diabetes). The insulin my body produces was inadequate. If your A1C is getting close to the 7.0% you need to start asking what is going on and changing what you eat. Without changing something, I was doomed.

Most people hide the fact that they are fighting diabetes and will not talk about their struggles; it is a great secret. I was never aware of the dangers that having diabetes can cause, but my A1C had been climbing higher for the last twenty years. I have been trying to control it with my diet and was told by most of my doctors that I need to start eating better, but all they ever told me was eat less sugar or use sugar alternatives. Some would tell us to use less salt and stop eating eggs, meat, and pork. Some said quit eating hamburgers and steaks, and do not eat bacon. We were told to buy margarine that was better in helping lower your cholesterol level and eat more fruits and vegetables. I remember hearing an apple a day keeps the doctor away. In the last five years or so, the guidelines for allowable blood glucose levels have gone up, making people feel that they are still in safe levels.

Now into my seventies, I have not had many daily blood glucose readings under two hundred. I have been doing my own A1C testing here at home for ten years and have seen what I was eating was making it worse. When I did my last A1C test, I was concerned it was too high, so I had my checkup and had to wait a few days for the results. I was still hoping it was not bad as we drove home. However, that A1C number was shocking to hear over the phone; it was now 10.0, and I needed to come to town to learn how to give myself a shot. Well, that was not happening because I was not going to be dependent on a shot that I would need forever.

My brand-new struggle with diabetes had begun. I started eating eggs and longhorn cheese and drinking water every meal for weeks. After three weeks, I did my A1C and it was down to 9.2. Well, I knew I could beat this; I just needed to find some other things I could eat. I came into the living room, got on YouTube, and searched for foods that I could eat with my high readings. I found a doctor that made many videos about this problem. In the video I watched, he explained that carbohydrates were the reason for my high levels. He said to stop all sugars and drop your carbs down to thirty or less a day.

Well, after doing what he advised, in two weeks, my A1C was down to 8.5. I have been looking for foods with less than one or zero carbs.

We have been buying things made of almond flour and using Stevia to sweeten things that need it. It was another six weeks, and my A1C was 7.7. My diet had been at three or less carbs a day for the last five weeks, and my lowest reading so far was 7.2. During my three-months' struggle, I lost twenty pounds. At this time, I have lost ninety pounds since I retired from the coal mine in February 2012. I am now just a few pounds from reaching my normal weight.

Well, you might wonder how all this happened. The reason I found myself in such an extreme A1C level was because I knew nothing about getting older and eating carbohydrates. My motivation for getting my body back to normal levels has always been to never let Lawrence down. He has been the angel in our family that was dealt a bad hand at birth but has achieved so many wonderful things anyway. As I am writing this, I have just ended my three-month waiting period for my 10.0 test. My A1C is 6.8. I thank my doctor, who takes care of all of us and for her patience and understanding through these exciting three months. She told me that all she needs to do is threaten me with a shot. She cut back on metformin and blood pressure medicine, and no shots or extra meds needed. I'm just winning a battle for Lawrence, and I am planning to be here for him as long as he needs me.

Thank you, Jesus, for giving me guidance and keeping me alive.

ACKNOWLEDGMENTS

First, I would like to thank Jesus!

I would like to thank all the people that have interacted with me in my lifetime, with first my parents, Red and Nina Waldie, and Judy's mother, Janie Barton,

Thanks to all my wonderful relatives and friends that have both laughed and cried with us through the years.

Thank you to all the people I worked with and the ones I worked for in the uranium mining industry, the coal mine, and the trucking business. Even my challenging foreman at the coal mine I am glad to call my friend.

Thank you to all the volunteers I have worked with in my life who built the Uranium Capital Bi-County Fair Grounds and Rodeo Grounds. You are all friends of mine forever.

And one special friend, Kathy, thank you for always being there to look after things when we were taking Lawrence on RV trips to see Jeremy.

I want to especially thank Lawrence's older brother and protector for many years, Jeremy, and his lovely wife Adela and our favorite grandkids: Lucas, Sammy, and Emma.

But most important of all…

Thank you, Judy and Lawrence, for all the love, care, and inspiration you both have given to me and to everyone you ever met. I have been super proud of getting to fight this battle with you guys and I will never, never give up.

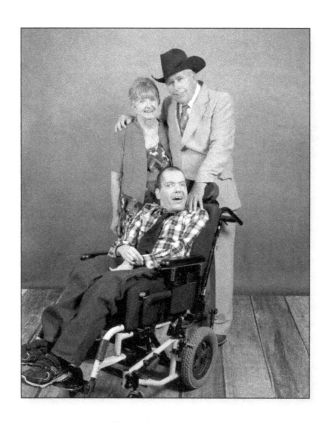

Rollie, Judy, and Lawrence

Thank you to Ken Brown Photography for the photographic work.

Printed in the USA
CPSIA information can be obtained
at www.ICGtesting.com
LVHW041327141023
760904LV00007B/797